A comprehensive guide on overall wellness after prostate cancer diagnosis

Empowering Strategies and Insights for Thriving Through your Prostate Cancer Journey

By

Dr. Meghan .R. Stribling

Table of contents

About the book

Prostate Cancer Solution Guide: Empowering Understanding and Action

Prostate cancer affects millions worldwide, making awareness and education crucial in navigating its complexities. This comprehensive solution guide aims to equip individuals, families, and caregivers with essential knowledge to effectively combat this disease.

1. **Understanding Prostate Cancer**: The guide delves into the fundamentals of prostate cancer, elucidating its causes, risk factors, and stages. Explaining the intricate biological mechanisms involved, it provides clarity on how this cancer develops and progresses, empowering readers with a deeper understanding.

2. **Diagnostic Techniques and Early Detection**: Emphasizing the importance of early detection, the guide sheds light on various diagnostic methods available.

From PSA (ProstateSpecific Antigen) tests to advanced imaging technologies like MRI, it educates on the tools that aid in timely identification, potentially increasing treatment success rates.

3. **Treatment Options and Innovations**: Navigating treatment choices can be overwhelming. This guide presents a comprehensive overview of conventional treatments such as surgery, radiation, and chemotherapy. Additionally, it explores emerging therapies like immunotherapy and targeted treatments, highlighting their potential and current research status.

4. **Holistic Care and Lifestyle Strategies**: Beyond medical interventions, the guide emphasizes holistic care. It discusses the role of nutrition, exercise, and mental wellbeing in complementing traditional treatments, promoting overall health and resilience during prostate cancer journeys.

5. **Navigating Support Systems**: Recognizing the emotional toll of a prostate cancer diagnosis, the guide addresses the importance of support networks. It offers guidance on finding support groups, counseling services, and resources to assist both patients and their loved ones throughout the treatment process.

In essence, the Prostate Cancer Solution Guide is a beacon of information and support, fostering empowerment through knowledge and resources for individuals confronting this challenge. Armed with insights from this guide, individuals can approach prostate cancer with informed decision making and a comprehensive approach towards health and healing.

Foreword

In a world where medical breakthroughs seem like distant hopes, there emerged a beacon of promise against the ominous threat of prostate cancer. Meet Dr. Meghan .R. Stribling a brilliant oncologist whose fervent dedication sparked a revolution in cancer treatment. His journey began amidst the staggering statistics that painted prostate cancer as a formidable adversary, silently affecting millions of lives.

Driven by a relentless pursuit of a solution, she embarked on a quest that intertwined groundbreaking research with unwavering determination. Years of meticulous study and tireless experimentation led him to develop a novel approach—nanotechnology infused with immunotherapy. It was a fusion of cutting edge science and compassionate innovation.

The breakthrough lay in the nanobots, minuscule marvels engineered to seek out and precisely target cancerous cells in the prostate. These microscopic warriors, armed with therapeutic payloads, navigated the intricate pathways of the human body, delivering a precise, lethal blow to the malignant growth without harming healthy tissues.

However Dr. Meghan .R. Stribling
encountered formidable obstacles along the way. Skepticism from peers and funding challenges threatened to stall his progress. Yet, his unwavering belief in the potential of his discovery propelled him forward. With the support of a dedicated team, he persevered, surmounting every hurdle through sheer resilience and a fervent desire to alleviate the suffering caused by prostate cancer.

Finally, after years of tenacious effort, rigorous trials, and unyielding dedication,.Dr. Meghan .R. Stribling
emerged triumphant. The once elusive solution to prostate cancer stood within reach, offering hope where there was once despair. The fusion of nanotechnology and immunotherapy stood poised to revolutionize cancer treatment, marking a pivotal moment in the fight against this formidable disease.

Chapter 1

Introduction to Prostate Cancer

1.1 Understanding Prostate Cancer

Prostate cancer, a prevalent malignancy among men globally, originates in the prostate gland—a vital component of the male reproductive system. The gland, situated beneath the bladder and anterior to the rectum, is susceptible to the development of cancerous cells. Often, this cancer progresses slowly and remains asymptomatic in its initial stages, underscoring the significance of regular screenings for timely detection and effective intervention.

Several risk factors contribute to the likelihood of prostate cancer. Advanced age, familial history, and racial predispositions markedly heighten susceptibility. Men over 50 face an increased risk, with the majority of diagnoses occurring in this age group. Additionally, a family history of prostate cancer amplifies the likelihood of its occurrence, indicating a genetic inclination. Moreover, African American men exhibit a higher vulnerability to aggressive forms of prostate cancer compared to other ethnicities.

Understanding the intricate pathophysiology of prostate cancer poses an ongoing challenge. Researchers continually explore hormonal, genetic, and environmental influences contributing to the transformation of normal prostate cells into cancerous ones. This complexity hampers the development of more effective treatment modalities and preventive measures.

Timely detection significantly influences treatment outcomes. Screening methods, including the prostate specific antigen (PSA) test and digital rectal examination (DRE), offer insights into potential cancer presence. A conclusive diagnosis often requires a biopsy, analyzing tissue samples microscopically.

Treatment approaches vary based on cancer stage, patient health, and preferences. Active surveillance, surgery, radiation therapy, hormone therapy, chemotherapy, or combinations thereof constitute potential treatments. Advanced therapies and targeted treatments continue to reshape prostate cancer care, fostering optimism for improved survival rates and reduced adverse effects.

Understanding prostate cancer's intricacies—risk factors, diagnosis, and treatments—is pivotal for patients, caregivers, and healthcare providers. Enhanced awareness, coupled with ongoing research endeavors, is key to combating this disease and enhancing the lives of affected individuals.

1.2 Risk Factors and Causes

Prostate cancer develops when cells in the prostate gland grow abnormally. Several risk factors and causes contribute to the development of this disease.

Age is a primary risk factor for prostate cancer. The likelihood of developing it increases with age, especially in men over 50. Genetics also play a role; having a family history of prostate cancer increases the risk, particularly if a close relative like a father or brother had the disease.

Ethnicity is another factor. African American men have a higher risk of developing prostate cancer compared to men of other races. The reasons for this higher risk are not entirely clear but could involve genetic, environmental, or lifestyle factors.

Certain genetic mutations or inherited gene changes, such as BRCA1 and BRCA2, usually associated with breast cancer in women, may also increase the risk of prostate cancer in men.

Dietary habits and lifestyle choices contribute to prostate cancer risk. High intake of red meat or high fat dairy products and a diet low in fruits and vegetables may elevate the risk. Obesity is linked to a higher likelihood of aggressive forms of prostate cancer.

Exposure to certain environmental factors and chemicals may play a role. Occupational exposure to cadmium, Agent Orange, or other pesticides might increase the risk, though the direct impact requires further research.

Inflammation or prostatitis (inflammation of the prostate) could potentially elevate the risk or contribute to the development of prostate cancer, but the exact relationship between the two is still under investigation.

Overall, while these factors can increase the likelihood of developing prostate cancer, many cases occur in men without any apparent risk factors, indicating the complexity and multifactorial nature of the disease. Regular screenings, a balanced diet, maintaining a healthy weight, and discussing individual risk factors with a healthcare professional are essential steps for managing and potentially reducing the risk of prostate cancer.

Chapter 2

Diagnosis and Detection

2.1 Screening for Prostate Cancer

Prostate cancer screening aims to detect the disease early, even before symptoms manifest, to improve the chances of successful treatment. The two primary screening methods for prostate cancer are the prostate specific antigen (PSA) blood test and digital rectal exam (DRE).

The PSA test measures the levels of a protein produced by the prostate gland in the blood. Elevated PSA levels can indicate various prostate issues, including cancer, but not all cases of elevated PSA lead to cancer. It's essential to interpret PSA levels alongside other factors, such as age, family history, and overall health.

The DRE involves a doctor inserting a lubricated, gloved finger into the rectum to feel the prostate gland's size, shape, and texture. Changes or abnormalities in the gland might suggest the presence of cancer.

Discussing the benefits and limitations of screening with a healthcare professional is crucial. While these tests can help detect prostate cancer early, they can also lead to false positives, unnecessary biopsies, and potential overdiagnosis or overtreatment. Shared decision making between the patient and healthcare provider regarding screening frequency and individual risk factors is vital for informed choices about prostate cancer screening.

2.2 Diagnostic Tests and Procedures

Diagnostic tests and procedures play a pivotal role in identifying and confirming various health conditions, including prostate cancer. For prostate cancer diagnosis, several key methods are employed:

1. **Biopsy**: This is the gold standard for confirming prostate cancer. It involves the removal of a small tissue sample from the prostate gland for examination under a microscope. A biopsy can determine the presence of cancer cells, their aggressiveness, and help guide treatment decisions.

2. .**Imaging Tests:** Imaging techniques like MRI (Magnetic Resonance Imaging), CT (Computed Tomography) scans, and ultrasound may be used to visualize the prostate gland and detect any abnormalities or potential tumors. These tests provide detailed pictures of the

prostate to aid in diagnosis and staging of the cancer.

3. **.PSA Test:.** While primarily a screening tool, the prostate specific antigen (PSA) blood test can also help in diagnosis. Elevated PSA levels may prompt further investigation, but it's not definitive for diagnosing prostate cancer; a biopsy is usually needed for confirmation.

4. **Digital Rectal Exam (DRE)**: Though primarily a screening tool, a DRE can also provide some diagnostic information. Abnormalities in the size, shape, or texture of the prostate gland felt during this exam might indicate the presence of cancerous growths.

These diagnostic methods are often used together to provide a comprehensive understanding of a potential prostate cancer diagnosis. Biopsy remains the most definitive way to confirm the presence of cancer cells. These tests, combined with a thorough medical history and physical examination, assist healthcare professionals in accurately diagnosing and staging prostate cancer, enabling them to create a tailored treatment plan for each patient.

Chapter 3

Stages and Grading

3.1 Staging of Prostate Cancer

Staging in prostate cancer refers to determining the extent and spread of the disease. It helps healthcare professionals understand how advanced the cancer is, guiding treatment decisions and predicting the outlook for the patient. The most commonly used staging system for prostate cancer is the TNM system:

1. .**Tumor (T)**: This indicates the size and extent of the primary tumor within the prostate gland. It ranges from T1 (where the tumor can't be felt or seen on imaging) to T4 (where the tumor has spread beyond the prostate).

2. **Node (N)**: This describes whether the cancer has spread to nearby lymph nodes. The scale ranges from N0 (no

lymph node involvement) to N1 (cancer detected in nearby lymph nodes).

3. **Metastasis (M):.** This denotes whether the cancer has spread to distant parts of the body. M0 indicates no distant spread, while M1 signifies metastasis to other organs like bones, lungs, or liver.

Combining these factors provides an overall stage grouping from I to IV, indicating the extent and severity of the cancer. Lower stages (I and II) typically denote localized cancer, while higher stages (III and IV) indicate more advanced or metastatic disease.

Accurate staging assists in determining appropriate treatment options, including surgery, radiation, hormone therapy, chemotherapy, or other targeted therapies. Staging also helps in predicting prognosis and guiding followup care to manage and monitor the disease effectively.

3.2 Gleason Score and Grading

The Gleason score and grading system are crucial in understanding the aggressiveness and severity of prostate cancer.

1. **Gleason Score**: It's a grading system used after examining prostate tissue samples obtained through biopsy. Pathologists assign a Gleason score based on how closely the cancer cells resemble normal prostate cells. The score ranges from 6 to 10:

Scores of 6 or lower (Gleason Grade Group 1) indicate well differentiated and less aggressive cancer cells.

Scores between 7 (Grade Group 2 or 3) suggest moderately differentiated cells with some aggressive characteristics.

Scores of 8 to 10 (Grade Groups 4 and 5) represent poorly differentiated and more aggressive cancer cells.

2. **Grading**: The Gleason grading system involves looking at two primary patterns of cancer cells within the prostate tissue sample. Each pattern is given a grade (ranging from 1 to 5), and the sum of these grades forms the Gleason score.

The first number represents the grade of the most common cancer cells observed.

The second number represents the grade of the next most prevalent cancer cells.

For instance, if a sample shows a primary pattern of 3 and a secondary pattern of 4, the Gleason score is 7 (3 + 4). The higher the Gleason score, the more aggressive the cancer is likely to be.

Understanding the Gleason score helps in determining the risk and aggressiveness of prostate cancer, guiding treatment decisions. Lower scores may indicate slower growing and less aggressive cancer, while higher scores suggest a more aggressive disease that may require more intensive treatment.

Chapter 4.

Treatment Options

4.1 Active Surveillance

Active surveillance is a strategy used to manage low risk prostate cancer without immediate aggressive treatment. It involves closely monitoring the cancer through regular checkups, PSA tests, biopsies, and imaging, rather than opting for immediate surgery or radiation.

Candidates for active surveillance typically have low grade and localized prostate cancer, meaning the cancer cells are less aggressive and contained within the prostate gland. The goal is to avoid potential side effects of immediate treatment, such as incontinence or erectile dysfunction, which may significantly impact quality of life.

During active surveillance:

1. .**Regular Monitoring**:. Patients undergo periodic examinations, PSA tests, and sometimes repeat biopsies to track any changes in the cancer's behavior or growth.

2. **Evaluation and DecisionMaking**:. If there's an increase in PSA levels or changes in biopsy results suggesting the cancer is becoming more aggressive, the healthcare team might recommend transitioning to active treatment.

3. .**Lifestyle and Followup Care**:. Patients are advised on lifestyle modifications like diet and exercise to support overall health. Regular followup visits and discussions with healthcare providers are essential to assess any changes and discuss further steps.

Active surveillance does not mean ignoring cancer; rather, it involves active monitoring to intervene if the cancer shows signs of progression. It allows patients to delay or potentially avoid treatment unless necessary, preserving their quality of life while ensuring timely intervention if the cancer becomes more aggressive. This approach is particularly suitable for older patients or those with other health conditions who might be at higher risk for complications from aggressive treatments.

4.2 Surgery (Prostatectomy)

Surgery, specifically prostatectomy, is a common treatment for prostate cancer. It involves the surgical removal of the prostate gland and surrounding tissues where the cancer is localized. There are different types of prostatectomy:

1. **Radical Prostatectomy:.** This procedure involves removing the entire prostate gland along with nearby tissues, including seminal vesicles. It can be done through different approaches: open surgery (with a large incision),

laparoscopic surgery (using small incisions and specialized tools), or robot assisted laparoscopic surgery (where a surgeon controls robotic arms to perform the operation).

2. **.Pelvic Lymph Node Dissection:.** In some cases, surgeons may also remove nearby lymph nodes to check for cancer spread.

After surgery:

1. **Recovery**:. Recovery time varies, but patients may need to stay in the hospital for a few days. It takes weeks to months to fully recover and resume normal activities.

2. **Potential Side Effects:.** Common side effects include urinary incontinence and erectile dysfunction. However, advancements in surgical techniques aim to minimize these side effects.

3. **.Followup Care:** Patients require regular followup appointments and monitoring,

including PSA tests, to ensure the cancer has been successfully removed and does not recur.

Surgery is most suitable for localized prostate cancer and is often recommended for younger, healthier patients with longer life expectancies. The goal is to remove the cancerous tissue entirely, potentially curing the cancer and preventing its spread to other parts of the body. Discussing the benefits, risks, and potential side effects with a healthcare provider is crucial in making an informed decision about undergoing prostatectomy.

4.3. Radiation Therapy

Radiation therapy is a common treatment for prostate cancer, aiming to kill cancer cells or prevent their growth using high energy rays. There are two primary types of radiation therapy used for prostate cancer:

1. **.External Beam Radiation Therapy (EBRT):.** This involves directing radiation beams from outside the body

toward the prostate gland. Modern EBRT techniques, such as IntensityModulated Radiation Therapy (IMRT) or Stereotactic Body Radiation Therapy (SBRT), precisely target the cancer while minimizing damage to surrounding healthy tissues.

2. .**Brachytherapy**:. In this approach, tiny radioactive seeds or pellets are implanted directly into the prostate. These seeds emit radiation that targets the cancer cells while minimizing exposure to nearby healthy tissues.

Radiation therapy can be used as the primary treatment for localized prostate cancer or in combination with other treatments, such as surgery or hormone therapy, depending on the cancer's stage and individual patient factors.

After radiation therapy:

1. .**Side Effects:**. Common side effects may include fatigue, urinary problems (such as frequency, urgency, or discomfort), bowel changes, and erectile dysfunction.

These side effects may vary based on the type and dosage of radiation used.

2. .**Followup Care:.** Regular followup visits with healthcare providers are essential to monitor for any potential recurrence or long term side effects. PSA tests and imaging may be performed to track the cancer's response to treatment.

Radiation therapy aims to effectively treat prostate cancer while preserving as much normal tissue function as possible. It's a valuable treatment option, especially for patients who may not be suitable candidates for surgery or those who prefer a noninvasive approach. Discussing the benefits, risks, and potential side effects with a healthcare provider helps in making an informed decision about undergoing radiation therapy for prostate cancer.

4.4 Hormone Therapy

Hormone therapy, also known as androgen deprivation therapy (ADT), is a treatment for prostate cancer that aims to lower the levels of male hormones, specifically testosterone, which can fuel the growth of prostate cancer cells.

How it works:

1. .**Testosterone Suppression**:. Prostate cancer cells often rely on testosterone to grow and spread. Hormone therapy disrupts this by either blocking the production of testosterone in the testes or interfering with the hormone's ability to stimulate cancer cells.

2. .**Types of Hormone Therapy**:. There are different methods to achieve testosterone suppression:

    - **Medications**: These drugs, known as LHRH agonists or antagonists, work on the pituitary gland to reduce testosterone production.

- **Antiandrogens**: These drugs block the action of androgens, including testosterone, from reaching the cancer cells.

- **Orchiectomy**: Surgical removal of the testicles, the main source of testosterone, is another way to reduce hormone levels.

Hormone therapy can be used in various stages of prostate cancer:

As an initial treatment for advanced or metastatic prostate cancer.
As adjuvant therapy alongside other treatments like radiation to enhance their effectiveness.
As a palliative treatment to manage cancer that has spread and relieve symptoms.

Side effects of hormone therapy may include:

- Reduced libido or sexual function.

- Hot flashes.
- Fatigue.
- Loss of muscle mass or strength.
- Osteoporosis or bone thinning.

Hormone therapy is not a cure for prostate cancer but can effectively control the disease by slowing its progression or shrinking the tumor. It's often used in combination with other treatments and plays a crucial role in managing advanced prostate cancer. Discussing the potential benefits, side effects, and treatment goals with a healthcare provider is essential when considering hormone therapy for prostate cancer.

4.5. Chemotherapy

Chemotherapy is a treatment for prostate cancer that involves using drugs to destroy cancer cells or slow down their growth. Unlike some other cancer treatments that target specific areas, chemotherapy drugs circulate throughout the body, affecting cancer cells wherever they may be.

When it's used:

Chemotherapy is typically employed in more advanced stages of prostate cancer, especially when the cancer has spread to other parts of the body (metastatic prostate cancer).
It's often used when other treatments haven't been successful or when the cancer is aggressive and requires a systemic approach.

How it works:

Chemotherapy drugs work by interfering with the ability of rapidly dividing cancer cells to grow and multiply.

These drugs target not only cancer cells but also normal cells that divide quickly, which can lead to certain side effects.

Administering chemotherapy:

Chemotherapy for prostate cancer is usually given through an intravenous (IV) infusion or as oral medications.

It's typically given in cycles, with periods of treatment followed by breaks to allow the body to recover from side effects.

Side effects of chemotherapy may include:

- Fatigue
- Nausea and vomiting
- Hair loss
- Lowered blood cell counts (increasing the risk of infection or bleeding)
- Changes in appetite

Chemotherapy for prostate cancer may not cure the disease, especially in its advanced stages. However, it can help to shrink tumors, alleviate symptoms, and slow the cancer's progression, thereby improving a person's quality of life. It's often used in combination with other treatments, and the decision to undergo chemotherapy depends on various factors, including the stage and aggressiveness of the cancer, overall health, and treatment goals, and should be discussed thoroughly with a healthcare provider.

4.6 Immunotherapy

Immunotherapy is a type of treatment for prostate cancer that boosts the body's natural immune system to fight cancer cells. It involves using medications that stimulate the immune system or help it recognize and attack cancer cells more effectively.

How it works:

Immunotherapy for prostate cancer includes different approaches such as immune checkpoint inhibitors, therapeutic vaccines, and adoptive cell therapy.

1. Immune checkpoint inhibitors: These drugs block certain proteins that cancer cells use to evade the immune system, allowing the immune system to recognize and attack the cancer cells more effectively.

2. Therapeutic **vaccines:** These vaccines stimulate the immune system to recognize and target prostate cancer cells.

3. **Adoptive cell therapy:** This involves modifying a patient's immune cells in a laboratory to enhance their ability to attack cancer cells, then reinfusing them back into the patient's body.

Use in prostate cancer:

Immunotherapy has shown promise in certain cases of advanced prostate cancer, especially when other treatments may not be as effective.

It's often considered when the cancer has spread to other parts of the body (metastatic prostate cancer) or hasn't responded to other treatments.

Potential side effects:

Side effects of immunotherapy may include fatigue, skin reactions, flu like symptoms, and inflammation in various parts of the body. In some cases, immune related side effects affecting the lungs, intestines, or other organs may occur.

Immunotherapy represents a newer approach to treating prostate cancer. While it might not be suitable for every patient or every stage of the disease, ongoing research continues to explore and develop new immunotherapy options to enhance its effectiveness in fighting prostate cancer. As with any treatment, discussing the potential benefits, risks, and suitability of immunotherapy with a healthcare provider is essential.

Chapter 5

Managing Side Effect

5.1. Coping with Treatment Side Effects

Coping with treatment side effects during prostate cancer care is crucial for maintaining quality of life. Here are some simple strategies for managing common side effects:

1. **Urinary Problems**: Practice pelvic floor exercises (Kegel exercises) to strengthen urinary control.Limit caffeine and alcohol intake, as they can irritate the bladder. Consult a healthcare provider for medications or techniques to manage urinary symptoms.

2. .**Erectile Dysfunction:** Discuss options like medications, vacuum erection devices, or implants with a healthcare provider to manage erectile dysfunction.

Openly communicate with your partner about intimacy concerns and explore alternative ways to maintain intimacy and closeness.

3. .**Fatigue**: Prioritize rest and sleep. Engage in gentle exercises like walking to combat fatigue.Plan activities throughout the day and conserve energy by taking breaks when needed.

4. **Bowel Changes:** Consume a high fiber diet with plenty of fluids to prevent constipation. Avoid foods that might irritate the digestive system and consider over the counter remedies under healthcare provider guidance.

5. **Hot Flashes:** Dress in layers to easily adjust clothing according to body temperature. Try relaxation techniques like deep breathing or meditation to manage hot flashes.

6. **Emotional Support:**Seek support from family, friends, or support groups to talk about concerns and emotions related to

treatment side effects.Consider counseling or therapy to help manage stress and anxiety.

7. **Healthy Lifestyle**: Maintain a balanced diet rich in fruits, vegetables, and lean proteins to support overall health during treatment. Stay physically active within your capabilities to improve energy levels and mood.

It's essential to communicate openly with healthcare providers about any side effects experienced during prostate cancer treatment. They can offer guidance, medications, or additional support to help manage these side effects effectively. Engaging in self care practices and seeking support from loved ones or professionals can significantly contribute to coping with treatment related challenges.

5.2 Supportive Care and Lifestyle Changes

Supportive care and lifestyle changes are integral parts of managing prostate cancer, focusing on improving overall wellbeing and aiding treatment effectiveness. Here are simple strategies:

1. **Healthy Eating**:. Consume a balanced diet rich in fruits, vegetables, whole grains, and lean protein. Limit intake of processed foods, saturated fats, and sugars to maintain a healthy weight and support the body's immune system.

2. .**Physical Activity:**Engage in regular physical activity tailored to your abilities, such as walking, swimming, or gentle exercises, to boost energy levels and maintain muscle strength.

3. **Stress Management:** Practice stress relief techniques like deep breathing, meditation, yoga, or mindfulness to

reduce anxiety and improve mental wellbeing.

4. **.Quit Smoking and Limit Alcohol:.**Quit smoking to reduce cancer related risks and improve overall health Limit alcohol consumption, as excessive drinking can negatively impact health and increase cancer risks.

5. **Support Networks:.** Seek support from family, friends, or support groups to share experiences and find emotional support.Consider joining prostate cancer support groups for information and camaraderie.

6. **Follow Medical Advice:.**Adhere to treatment plans and attend regular checkups and screenings as recommended by healthcare providers. Communicate openly with healthcare professionals about any concerns or changes in health during and after treatment.

7. .**Manage Side Effects:** Take medications as prescribed and discuss any side effects experienced with healthcare providers. Explore supportive therapies like acupuncture or massage to alleviate treatment related discomfort.

8. .**Quality Sleep:.**Maintain a consistent sleep schedule and create a relaxing bedtime routine to improve sleep quality and overall health.

Adopting a healthy lifestyle and seeking supportive care not only supports the body during prostate cancer treatment but also contributes to improved physical and emotional wellbeing. These lifestyle changes can complement medical treatments, enhance resilience, and positively impact overall health outcomes. Always consult healthcare providers before making significant lifestyle changes during cancer treatment.

Chapter 6

Clinical Trials and Research

6.1 Exploring New Treatments and Innovations

Exploring new treatments and innovations for prostate cancer involves ongoing research and advancements aimed at improving outcomes and expanding treatment options. Here are key aspects in simple terms:

1. **Precision Medicine:.** Researchers are studying genetic and molecular factors to develop targeted therapies that specifically focus on cancer cells while minimizing damage to healthy cells. This approach aims to create personalized treatments based on an individual's unique genetic makeup and the characteristics of their cancer.

2. **.Immunotherapy Advancements:.** Ongoing research explores ways to enhance the effectiveness of immunotherapy for prostate cancer by developing new drugs and combination therapies. This includes investigating different types of immune checkpoint inhibitors, vaccines, and adoptive cell therapies.

3. **Advances in Radiation Therapy:.** Innovative techniques in radiation therapy, such as proton therapy and stereotactic body radiation therapy (SBRT), aim to deliver precise radiation doses to the tumor while reducing exposure to surrounding healthy tissues. These advancements potentially improve treatment outcomes and minimize side effects.

4. **Clinical Trials:.** Researchers conduct clinical trials to test new treatments, drugs, or combinations of therapies. These trials provide opportunities for patients to access innovative treatments that are still under investigation and

contribute to advancing prostate cancer care.

5. **Liquid Biopsies:.** Scientists are exploring liquid biopsies, which involve analyzing blood or urine samples to detect genetic material or cancer cells shed by tumors. This noninvasive method could provide insights into cancer progression, treatment response, and the development of targeted therapies.

6. **Artificial Intelligence** (AI) and Imaging:. imaging techniques aim to improve early detection, accurate diagnosis, and monitoring of prostate cancer. These innovations enhance the precision of imaging tools, aiding in treatment planning and assessment.

Continued research and innovation in prostate cancer treatment offer hope for improved outcomes, reduced side effects, and personalized therapies tailored to individual patients. Participation in clinical trials and staying informed about emerging treatments can provide opportunities for accessing cutting edge treatments and contributing to the advancement of prostate cancer care.

6.2 Understanding Clinical Trials

Understanding clinical trials in simple terms involves knowing the purpose, process, and potential benefits of these research studies for prostate cancer:

1. **Purpose**:. Clinical trials are research studies designed to evaluate new treatments, drugs, procedures, or interventions to improve prostate cancer care. They aim to test the safety, effectiveness, and potential side effects of these innovations.

2. **Types of Trials:**.

- Treatment Trials:. Test new treatments or combinations of treatments for prostate cancer.
- Prevention Trials:. Evaluate ways to prevent prostate cancer or its recurrence.
- Screening Trials:. Study new methods for detecting prostate cancer at earlier stages.
- Quality of Life Trials:. Focus on improving the comfort and quality of life for individuals living with prostate cancer.

3. .**Phases of Clinical Trials**:. Trials go through different phases:
- Phase I:. Initial testing to determine safety and dosage.
- Phase II:. Assessing effectiveness and further safety.
- Phase III:. Comparing new treatments to standard treatments for efficacy, safety, and side effects.
- Phase IV:. Post Marketing studies after a treatment is approved to monitor long term safety and effectiveness.

4. **Participant Involvement:.** Individuals who participate in clinical trials play a vital role in advancing prostate cancer treatments. Participants receive either the experimental treatment or the standard treatment (or a placebo) and are closely monitored by healthcare professionals throughout the trial.

5. **.Benefits and Risks**:. Clinical trials offer potential benefits such as access to new treatments, contributing to medical knowledge, and receiving expert care. However, there are potential risks, including unknown side effects and uncertainty about the treatment's effectiveness.

6. **Informed Consent:.** Before joining a trial, participants receive detailed information about the trial, including its purpose, procedures, risks, and benefits. They voluntarily provide informed consent after understanding the information.

Clinical trials are crucial for advancing prostate cancer treatments and improving patient outcomes. Participating in these trials can provide access to innovative therapies and contribute to the development of better treatments for prostate cancer. Individuals considering participation in clinical trials should discuss the options thoroughly with healthcare providers to make informed decisions about their involvement.

7 Conclusion

7.1 simple strategies for preventing prostate cancer:

1. **Healthy Diet:.** Consume a balanced diet rich in fruits, vegetables, whole grains, and lean proteins. Limit intake of processed foods, saturated fats, and sugars.

2. **.Regular Exercise:.** Engage in regular physical activity, such as brisk walking, jogging, or cycling, for at least 30 minutes most days of the week.

3. **.Maintain a Healthy Weight:.** Aim to achieve and maintain a healthy weight by adopting a balanced diet and staying physically active.

4. **Limit Alcohol:.** Moderate alcohol consumption, or consider avoiding it

altogether, as excessive drinking is linked to increased cancer risks.

5. .**Stop Smoking**:. Quit smoking, as smoking is associated with a higher risk of developing aggressive forms of prostate cancer.

6. **Annual Checkups**:. Regular medical checkups and screenings for prostate cancer, especially for men over 50, can help detect the disease early when it's more treatable.

7. **Consider Supplements**:. Discuss with a healthcare provider about the potential benefits of specific supplements like vitamin D or selenium, which may have a protective effect against prostate cancer.

8. **Healthy Lifestyle Choices**:. Prioritize a healthy lifestyle by managing stress, getting adequate sleep, and avoiding exposure to environmental toxins or chemicals.

adopting a healthy lifestyle and making informed choices can potentially reduce the risk of developing the disease. Discussing prevention strategies with a healthcare provider can provide personalized guidance based on individual health factors and family history.

7.2. Prognosis and Long Term Outlook

Understanding the prognosis and long term outlook for prostate cancer involves considering several factors:

1. **.Stage of Cancer:.** The stage at which prostate cancer is diagnosed plays a significant role in determining the long term outlook. Early Stage cancers confined to the prostate often have better prognosis compared to cancers that have spread to other parts of the body.

2. **Gleason Score:.** The Gleason score, which indicates the aggressiveness of the cancer cells, helps predict how quickly

the cancer may grow and spread. Lower Gleason scores (6 or below) usually indicate a less aggressive cancer with better long term outcomes.

3. **Treatment Response:.** The response to treatments like surgery, radiation, chemotherapy, hormone therapy, or immunotherapy influences the long term outlook. Successful treatment that effectively controls or eliminates the cancer can positively impact prognosis.

4. **.PSA Levels**:. Prostate Specific antigen (PSA) levels after treatment can indicate how well the treatment has worked. A decrease or stabilization of PSA levels suggests a positive response to treatment.

5. **Overall Health:.** A patient's overall health, age, and any other existing medical conditions can affect the long term outlook. Generally, healthier individuals tend to respond better to treatment and have improved prognosis.

6. **Followup Care:.** Regular followup visits with healthcare providers for monitoring, including PSA tests and imaging, are crucial for tracking the cancer's response to treatment and detecting any potential recurrence or complications early.

Overall, the long term outlook for prostate cancer varies widely among individuals and depends on multiple factors. Many men diagnosed with early stage prostate cancer have excellent long term survival rates, while those with more advanced stages might require ongoing treatments and monitoring. Discussing prognosis and long term outlook with a healthcare provider, considering individual factors, can help individuals better understand their situation and make informed decisions about their prostate cancer journey.

Conclusion

In the journey of confronting prostate cancer, courage stands as an unwavering companion. The multifaceted approach delineated in "A Guide to Conquering Prostate Cancer with Courage" offers a beacon of hope amidst the complexities of this condition. This guide illuminates not just the medical intricacies but also the emotional fortitude necessary to navigate through the trials of prostate cancer.

Within these pages lies a roadmap, advocating for proactive screening, early detection, and diverse treatment modalities tailored to individual needs. Emphasizing the significance of a comprehensive support network, the guide echoes the importance of mental resilience, fostering a positive mindset, and seeking solace in the embrace of family, friends, and support groups.

The collaborative efforts of medical advancements, innovative therapies, and the tireless dedication of healthcare professionals converge in this guide, presenting an arsenal against prostate cancer. From conventional treatments like surgery and radiation to emerging approaches such as immunotherapy and targeted therapies, the spectrum of options detailed here offers a glimmer of optimism in the fight against this disease.

Furthermore, the guide extends beyond treatment strategies, highlighting lifestyle modifications, nutrition, and exercise as pivotal components in managing and preventing prostate cancer. It underscores the power of holistic wellbeing in augmenting the efficacy of medical interventions.

As this guide draws to a close, its underlying message persists—a resilient spirit bolstered by courage is the cornerstone in confronting prostate cancer. With knowledge as a weapon, courage as a shield, and unwavering support as armor, individuals facing prostate cancer can navigate this formidable terrain with steadfast determination and hope for a brighter, healthier tomorrow.

www.ingramcontent.com/pod-product-compliance
Lightning Source LLC
Chambersburg PA
CBHW071105260726
48661CB00006B/2476